Atkins Diet

The Ultimate Guide to Atkins Diet

Table of Contents

Introduction

I want to thank you and congratulate you for downloading *Atkins: Ultimate Guide to Atkins*!

Weight loss is something that nearly everyone struggles with, especially as we get older. As our metabolism slows down, it is much easier to gain fat, lose muscle, and face new health ailments that keep us from enjoying life. If you do a simple google search about how to lose weight, thousands of articles, diet plans, and workout routines will immediately pop up. Of course, the general idea for any weight loss plan is to eat right and exercise, right? So, out of the hundreds of methods you can choose from, which one is right for you?

Atkins has been proven to be the most efficient and effective weight loss plan out there. It has helped millions of people around the globe find health and happiness through its strict but effective regiment. The question is, how do you know if Atkins will work for you and give you the results you want? The answer is simple. Atkins works for everyone whose goal is to burn fat and become healthier. This method in particular works because it keeps you from consuming foods that have any form of sugar, so that your body burns pure fat for energy instead.

The modern diet is largely made up of carbohydrates and fats, which do not work well together and contribute to the development of several diseases. This guide will teach you everything you need to know about the Atkins diet, as well as how your body functions using basic macronutrients. Through carefully laid out steps and strategies, you will learn how to become truly independent from sugar addiction, cravings, and common factors that attribute to falling off the wagon and going back to your old eating habits.

Here is an inescapable fact: most people will fail in their weight loss attempts. More than sixty- percent of the people who create goals and want to become healthier are unsuccessful and stay unhappy with their bodies. This guide gives you all the information you could possibly need to not only be successful in your journey of losing weight, but also become an inspiration and role model for other individuals who aspire to greater health. Knowledge is your greatest advantage to any new goal, and this book will teach you the science behind the Atkins diet, how cutting out carbohydrates can save your life, and a complete twenty – one-day meal plan to get you through the first phase of the program.

If you do not develop your understanding of weight loss, you will spend years looking for "the secret" or "magic supplement" that doesn't exist.

Too many people look for the easiest way to get what they want, without acknowledging that the greatest success comes from a little struggle and a lot of willpower. Atkins is not just a dieting program, but the most trusted and effective strategy to burning fat and achieving your goals that you will ever find.

It's time for you to become an amazing and happier you. Think of all the things you will miss out on if you do not change your habits and lead a healthier life. Now is the time to take control of your lifestyle and change for the better. You *can* be skinner, toned, strong, and healthy; if you choose to be. It is time for you to begin your journey of transformation and rejuvenation. Good luck and enjoy!

Chapter 1: What is Atkins? The Game- Changing Weight Loss Plan

The theory of dieting has been around for as long as society has wanted a solution to their weight loss and health needs. There are dozens of cultures, religions, and countries around the world who all promote and live by different eating habits; all of which have their own benefits and disadvantages. The various lifestyles lead to the cultivation of hundreds of diet plans and programs that all promise to help you lose weight. An idea that was not often practiced in the twentieth century is now a multi- billion- dollar institution that promotes and feeds off of the public's insecurities and resolutions. However, it was not until recently that any of these methods were particularly effective.

We live in an age where food is accessible and cheap, which makes it easy to over eat and make poor choices with meals. Many diets share the same focus of cutting out calories, so that your body begins utilizing more calories than what you are intaking to create energy. This leads to less water weight and overall loss of fat, muscle, and water. The general foundation of this method works, but not to the fullest extent of what you truly want when changing your eating habits so drastically. Eating in a caloric deficit will allow you to lose weight, but it will not help you to keep the weight off for good. In fact, many diets often leave the participant hungry and craving sugar- loaded foods. After your body is starved of calories for so long, the individual experiences a great relapse and binges more than they have in the past. This leads to gaining back all of the weight that you just lost, and then some. The vicious cycle continues as another weight loss program is found and the individual picks up right where they initially began. Different diet, same concept.

The reality is that even though most diets are based off of cutting out calories, there is not much evidence that suggests doing so will manifest long- term success. Thus, the search for a diet that works on a different strategy for overall health and weight loss continues. This is where Atkins comes into play. What many have considered to be another fad diet, has brought success in the journey for long- term weight loss for anyone who has dared to take on the challenge of cutting out something other than calories from their diet. Atkins takes a more scientific approach to the theory of losing weight by analyzing how the modernized western diet has changed.

Today, we consume more carbohydrates than ever before and rely on bread and starch as staples for every meal. Cereal, pasta, and bread on consumed on a daily basis, which leads to the body storing more fat and living off the short bursts of energy that simple carbohydrates fuel. There is much to be said about how carbs and fats interact with your body's chemistry; however, that will be discussed in a later chapter.

The Atkins diet was made famous by physician Dr. Robert C. Atkins through is best- selling book that explained the diet in 1972. Since the release of his work, the Atkins diet has reached all four corners of the globe and inspired millions of people to look at weight loss with a different perspective. Many books and articles have reanalyzed and digested the diet time and time again, all with their own unique take on the matter. At first, the Atkins diet was deemed unhealthy and even confronted mainstream health authorities for their use of carbohydrates and saturated fat. However, there have been dozens of studies that have proven the many benefits that Atkins has to offer, despite what skeptics and critics may believe.

Atkins does not promote the idea of cutting out calories from your diet, but simple carbohydrates and sugar. This idea was entirely new, but proved successful for many. This is because when you reduce your carb intake and increase your protein intake, your appetite greatly subsides and end up consuming less calories without even realizing it. Diets that are high in carbohydrates leave your appetite satisfied for a short amount of time, as cravings and hunger pangs will ensue just an hour after eating. Atkins begins by completely cutting out carbs, and then slowly reintroducing complex carbohydrates once your body has learned how to run efficiently without unnecessary sugar. There are several rules and guidelines that are outlined throughout the diet, however the complete long- term alteration of one's eating habits encourages individuals view Atkins as a lifestyle change, rather than a short- term solution to losing weight.

The key to staying successful with Atkins is sticking to it, even after the first phase is over. You will experience cravings and even perhaps lapses of judgement, just like you would have with any other dieting program. However, Atkins does not encourage you to keep to a restrictive regiment for too long, and reintroduces foods that you love as you learn how to correctly consume them in relation to the high consumption of protein and fat that Atkins requires. Now, you may be wondering how you could possibly give up bread and other sugary foods that have become staples to your diet. Once you have completed the first phase of the program, you will crave those foods less and be able to enjoy small amounts later on as you progress through the program.

Atkins Phases Broken Down

Phase 1:

Phase one is designed to help your body detox from sugar and become reliant on protein and fat for energy instead of carbohydrates. During this stage, you will consume under twenty grams of carbohydrates each day for approximately two weeks. Throughout the extent of phase one, you will eat meals that are high in fat, protein, and count your carbs through vegetables, like leafy greens.

Phase one allows your metabolism to kick- start into weight loss mode. So, that you can reprogram the way your body utilizes macronutrients. This first part of the programs is often mistaken for the structure of the entire program, but this is an inaccurate judgement. While you function off just twenty carbs a day, you begin understand the maximum grams of net carbs that you can eat while also experiencing weight loss and adequate energy levels. This is referred to as your personal carb balance, which will be established as you continue into the next phase.

This phase should last for a minimum of two weeks, although you can safely follow the guidelines of this phase for as long as you need to if your goal is to lose as much weight as possible in the shortest amount of time. In this case, you will continue with phase one until you are fifteen pounds away from your target weight.

Phase 2:

Once you have achieved your goal weight with phase one, it is time to begin phase two. During this part of the diet plan, the participant will slowly start to add in new types of carbohydrates. The purpose is to correctly reintroduce the right kind of carbohydrates into your meal plan, so that you are still giving your body the nutrients it needs while still losing weight. You will begin eating nuts, low- carb veggies, and small amounts of fruit; and you will continue this phase until you are within ten pounds of your target weight.

Keep in mind that just because you can start eating carbs again does not mean that you can eat whatever you want, as long as it isn't too much. Nuts, strawberries, melon, seeds, cottage cheese, blueberries, and cottage cheese are a few examples of what you are limited to during phase two. The purpose of adding some more carbohydrates to your meal in this phase is to help you keep your momentum that you gained in the beginning of phase one, while still attempting to find your personal carbohydrate balance. Although you may stay dedicated to phase two until you are within ten pounds of your target weight, you can transition into phase three sooner if you are willing to let your weight loss pace slow a little.

Phase 3:

Phase three marks the progress that you have made, as you are closer than ever to your target weight. At this point in the Atkins plan, you will add even more carbohydrates into your diet until your weight loss slightly slows down. This phase is meant to help you fine- tune your diet so that you can eventually focus on maintaining your weight loss when you come into phase four. During phase three, you will see how much you can increase your daily net carb consumption while still maintaining weight loss during while reintroducing a wider variety of carbohydrate- filled foods. You will remain in phase three until you have achieved your goal weight and maintained it for at least thirty days.

Phase 4:

Phase four is designed to help you maintain your weight loss and new health diet. During this part of the Atkins plan, you are allowed to consume as many health carbohydrates as your body can take without paying close attention to your weight. This phase is regarded as a lifetime lifestyle, when you generally stick with the meal plan as a long- term commitment; eating the same foods that you have already been consuming with each new phase. Some foods that you may have tried to reintroduce earlier on, your body can now adequately handle. As long as you maintain your target weight, you can continue experimenting with small amounts of different carbs and other foods that you enjoy.

The phases that mark the progression of the Atkin diet may seem a bit complicated or even unnecessary. However, the entire program is designed to help your body overcome the addiction to carbohydrates while still enjoying the tasty foods that you love. The truth of the matter is that you are the only one who fully understands how your body works. You will notice right away if part of the meal plan does not work for you and your needs, and can easily alter your strategy accordingly. While giving up carbohydrates for any length of time can prove to be challenging, the first phase only lasts for two weeks and the benefits of detoxing from sugar can last a lifetime.

Chapter 2: The Basics of Atkins

Efficient protein intake and working your body into a ketogenic state are critical components to maximizing fat loss and maintaining muscle during the Atkins diet. While the first phase of Atkins may require a minimum of two weeks of dedication, it will take approximately three weeks for your body to become adapted to its natural ketogenic function. During the beginning phase of Atkins, nitrogen loss may occur if your carb consumption is extremely low. This is due to the fact that when your carb intake decreases, your body resorts to converting protein into glucose. Approximately sixteen percent of protein is nitrogen, and thus the loss of muscle occurs and your metabolic rate will decrease. Issues like this arise when you are not consuming adequate amounts of protein. Although your body is used to converting carbohydrates into glucose for energy, it can efficiently do this with protein and fats as well. The reason that our bodies do not already default to this way of functioning is because the modern diet is largely made up of carbohydrates and sugary foods; which are easier to break down into glucose.

This issue is especially inconvenient for body builders and other gym goers, as building muscle is essential for their regiment. So, how many carbohydrates do you need in order to maintain muscle and spare protein loss? The greatest challenge that comes with limiting your carb intake is that your body can go into starvation mode for too long, which leads to muscle loss. Starvation mode occurs when you consume less than fifteen carbs per day; this is necessary for your body to utilize its fat stores for energy. When you increase your carb consumption to fifty grams per day, your body is less dependent on amino acids for glycogenesis. Glycogenesis occurs through two different mechanisms. Firstly, when the increased carb consumption results in high blood glucose and insulin levels, which restricts your cortisol release. And secondly, when the carbs supply the brain with glucose, inhibiting the breakdown of protein in the body.

While keeping to the Atkins diet, your overall protein intake should account for at least seventy – percent of your diet; with your fat intake making up twenty – percent, and carbohydrates accounting for the remaining ten percent. As you move into the second phase, your carb intake will increase by ten percent, as your fat and protein intake decrease slightly. As you continue through the program, you will slowly alter the percentage of your macronutrient intake as your body adjusts to the new meal plan.

You can easily figure out how many grams of protein, fat, and carbohydrates you should consume with each meal and on a daily basis by using online macronutrient calculators. The website will ask a variety of questions based on your goals and physical health in order to determine the correct macro proportions for your diet. You will have to fill in information regarding your:

- Age

- Weight
- Sex
- Height
- Daily or Weekly Activity Level
  - Sedentary
  - Lightly Active
  - Moderately Active
  - Very Active
- The Kind of Exercise You Typically Perform
- Current Body Fat Percentage
- Main Objective Regarding Your Diet
  - Lose Weight
  - Maintain Weight
  - Gain Muscle

What to Eat on the Atkins Diet?

Meat

- Bacon
- Beef
- Fish/ Seafood
- Poultry
- Pork
- Turkey

Eggs

Vegetables

- Artichokes
- Asparagus

- Broccoli
- Cabbage
- Celery
- Cauliflower
- Kale
- Lettuce
- Mushroom
- Onions
- Peppers
- Radishes
- Spinach
- Spaghetti Squash
- Zucchini

Fats/Oils

- Coconut
- Flaxseed
- Olive
- Sesame
- Sunflower

Dairy

- Butter
- Cheese
- Full Fat Cream Cheese
- Full Fat Yogurt
- Heavy Whipping Cream
- Sour Cream

Nuts and Seeds

(All nuts are permitted during Phases 2-4)

Seeds:

- Chia
- Flax
- Pumpkin
- Sesame
- Sunflower

Drinks

- Water
- Tea (Black)
- Coffee (Black)

Foods to Avoid While on the Atkins Diet

Breads and Grains

- Bagels
- Barley
- Couscous
- English Muffins
- Kaiser Rolls
- Oats
- Pasta
- Rice
- Tortillas
- Products Containing Flour
- Whole Grains

Vegetables (During Phase One Only)

- Beans
- Carrots
- Chickpeas

- Corn
- Hummus
- Lentils
- Peas
- Potatoes
- Soy Beans
- Tomatoes
- Turnips

Sweets

- Cake
- Cookies
- Ice Cream
- Pastries
- Pies
- Pudding
- Gelatin

Sugars and Sweeteners

- White Sugar
- Brown Sugar
- Sucralose
- Aspartame
- Erythritol
- Agave Nectar
- Xylitol

Drinks

- Alcohol
- Energy Drinks
- Hot Chocolate
- Juice

- Milk
- Protein Shakes
- Soft Drinks
- Sports Drinks
- Sweetened Teas

Vegetable Oils and Fats
- Canola Oil
- Vegetable Oil
- Soybean Oil
- Trans Fats

High – Carb Fruits
- Apples
- Bananas
- Grapes
- Oranges
- Pears

Adding Carbs Back into Your Diet After Phase One

Despite what many people may believe, the Atkins program is relatively flexible. The most difficult part of beginning this diet is the first phase, in which you will minimize your carb intake. Once the induction phase is over, you are allowed to slowly integrate healthy carbohydrates back into your diet. This includes vegetables that are higher in carbohydrates, fruits, starches, and healthy grains such as oats and brown rice. However, once you have made it to the final phase of the program, you will need to maintain that lifestyle for the long haul; even if you have achieved your weight loss and health goals.

It is crucial that you keep to the diet you have formed during the final phase because your body will react differently to the old foods that you used to eat. You may have bloating and trouble digesting as your body becomes sensitive to certain foods that may be difficult for it to process. Regardless, even if your body does not have a negative reaction to high carbohydrate food products, you will gain back the weight you lose during the last three phases. Of course, this rings true for any weight loss program you try.

Atkins allows you to eat the delicious foods you love, such as bacon and cheese. However, as you begin introducing new foods during the second phase, you can experiment with different types of carbohydrates. As your net carb intake increases to fifty grams, you can start eating dark chocolate, fruits, oats, etc. One of the most difficult factors for many people on this diet is finding foods to snack on. While you may not be able to go to your default bag of potato chips or candy, there are plenty of options to keep you satisfied with your salty and sweet cravings. Some examples of low – carb snacks include:

- Hard – boiled eggs
- Cheese
- Nuts and seeds
- Yogurt
- Berries and whipped cream
- Green tea

Chapter 3: The Science Behind the Diet: Why it Works

We have been lead to believe that the more carbs and less fat we have in our diets, the healthier we will be. After all, carbohydrates are a source of energy, while fat makes us fat. Right? Actually, this way of thinking is completely wrong. Our bodies are capable of many things, and one of them is converting fat and protein into energy. Why would you want to completely change your diet just so your body uses fat for energy? Because fat does not make you fat: sugar does. In fact, carbohydrates are made up of starch, fiber, and sugar. When broken down during the digestive process, the majority of these nutrients are stored away for later as fat. This means that the more carbohydrates you eat, the more your body will store away for later, as it only takes a small number of carbs to function on a day to day basis.

Fat, on the other hand, does not get stored away as fat cells when you consume too much of it; and neither does protein. When you cut out carbs from your diet and increase the amount of protein and fat you eat, the way your body functions entirely changes. Its traditional energy source is no longer available, so it must resort to using other nutrients for energy. When this happens, your body begins using your stored fat as fuel, and you begin to lose weight. This process is called ketosis.

Ketosis is something that your body does every day, whether you eat carbs or not. However, eating a low carb, high fat diet gives this process a natural boost. Your body breaks carbohydrates down into glucose, because glucose is needed to create energy. When your body does not have glucose to process, it goes into a deep state of ketosis. Your body will burn fat stores, creating molecules: ketones. Ketones occur when your body breaks down fat into fatty acids in the liver during a process known as beta- oxidation. Although during the first few weeks of ketosis, the individual will experience energy lulls, studies have shown that your body runs up to seventy percent more efficiently than when it uses glucose for energy. This coincides perfectly with our evolution as human beings. Our ancestors did not have access to the food that we eat today, and therefore relied on protein and fat to keep them nourished.

While your body is in ketosis, it is possible that it produces too many ketone bodies. Therefore, the body with naturally expel of excess ketones through urine. However, this is not a sign that your state of ketosis is slowing down, but that your brains has enough BHB (beta- hydroxybutyric acid) to keep functioning at a higher level. Although the idea of burning pure fat sounds great, your body does need glucose to maintain maximum health, which is why phase one is the only time during Atkins when you will severely limit your carb intake.

Your body can theoretically completely become independent from carbohydrates. This is due to the breakdown of excess protein in your diet. Protein can be used for energy, building muscle, and keeping your bones strong. However, when you eat too much protein, approximately fifty- six percent will be turned into glucose in the bloodstream. Therefore, it is crucial that you keep a strict eye on your protein intake during the first three phases; so you don't accidently knock your body out of ketosis.

It is important to recognize that ketosis and starvation are two entirely different things. Starvation occurs when your body has no source of food or nutrition. This will result in muscle loss as your body begins using its own stores of protein in your muscles to stay alive. Ketosis is a temporary state of fasting that will encourage your body to use some of your fat stores for energy to induce weight loss. When done correctly, the ketogenic process will preserve your muscle tissue.

What to Expect During Phase One: Introducing Your Body to Ketosis

When you start any diet, you will notice weight loss almost immediately. However, this "weight loss" is not stored fat, but simply water weight. The human body is mostly made up of water. When you consume a lot of carbohydrates, you may experience bloating, even the day after consuming a big meal. This is because carbohydrate molecules and water molecules cling to each other, resulting in excess water weight. During the beginning of the Atkins diet, you will first drop any bloating that is caused by retaining water.

Once your body has dropped its water weight, you will start to lose real pounds of fat. Although it is easy to get hung up on the scale, it is more important to note the more obvious physical changes. While you may only drop a few pounds when you weigh in, your waist may have shrunk by a few inches. Lost inches are relatively more significant than numbers on a scale. Your clothes will feel a bit looser even if the number on the scale does not budge. During the Atkins program, is it normal for your body to fluctuate on a daily basis. Keeping a constant eye on the scale is not an efficient way of measuring your progress on this diet.

Carbohydrate- filled foods often contain massive amounts of sodium, which is not necessarily a bad thing. As your body flushes out toxins, ketones, and other excess nutrients, it will begin to lose electrolytes as well. If you begin feeling ill or a lack of energy, try drinking full sodium broth every day. This technique will also stop constipation, headaches, and muscle cramps during the first phase.

The best way to begin the Atkins program is to lose any expectations you may have. Everyone's body is different, and will react in different ways to the sudden change in diet. Your friend may have lost seven pounds within the first week of phase one, but there is no way of knowing if you will lose the same amount. Just know that during induction, you are cleansing your body in the most efficient way, and becoming a better and healthier you with each passing day.

Chapter 4: Top Benefits of Cutting and Limiting Carbohydrates

Low carb- high fat diets have been used for thousands of years for its various healing benefits. Nearly every culture in the world recognizes some form of this program as a way to cure diseases, improve overall health, and enhance the body's natural functions. While weight loss may be your primary reason for switching to a ketogenic diet, there are other benefits that you should consider while making this transition.

1. Inhibiting Your Appetite (In a Positive Way)

Hunger is not only eventually leads to bingeing, but it is also possibly the worst side effect of dieting. Hunger is typically the main reason most people feel terrible while dieting and end up giving up on losing weight all together. Let's face it, no one likes hunger pangs. Possibly the best part about switching to a low-carb diet is the automatic reduction of your appetite. Various studies have shown that when cutting down carbs and increasing protein and fat intake, people end up eating much fewer calories than normal. Without even trying, you will already eat less than usual.

2. More Weight Loss Than You Expect

It is no secret that cutting out carbohydrates is the simplest and by far most effective method of losing weight. After learning the biological process of burning fat on the Atkins diet, it is easy to see that people on low- carb diets tend to lose more weight quicker than individuals who stick to a low- fat meal plan. Even when others may restrict calories, people who adopt a ketogenic diet will still have more success.

This is due, firstly, to the quick explement of excess water weight from the body. Additionally, due to lower insulin levels, your kidneys will also get rid of extra sodium through urination, resulting in even more weight loss. When comparing studies, experts have found that individuals who keep to a low carb diet will lose up to three times as much weight, without experiencing hunger.

The most successful weight loss stories featuring low- carb diets report sticking to the diet for longer than six months. This is because many people tend to resort back to their old eating habits after reaching their goal weight. This is why sticking with a low – carb diet as your lifestyle will create better results, as long-term commitment soon becomes second nature.

3. Most of the Fat Loss Achieved in from the Abdominal Cavity

Even though we all would love to lose fat from everywhere on our bodies, the reality is that not all fat in your body is the same. Where your fat is stored dictates how your health is affected and whether or not you are at risk for disease. Your body contains two kinds of fat: subcutaneous and visceral. Subcutaneous fat is the layer underneath your skin, while visceral fat resides in your abdominal cavity and around your organs. Too much visceral fat results in increased inflammation, insulin resistance, and metabolic dysfunction disorder; commonly found in Westernized countries.

Low- carb lifestyles are extremely effective at decreasing excess fat around your abdomen, so that stubborn belly fat is more likely to disappear during the first few phases of Atkins. The reduction of visceral fat will also reduce your potential of developing heart disease and type 2 diabetes.

4. Your Triglyceride Levels Will Drastically Decrease

Triglycerides are fat molecules. An excess of triglycerides is when there is high level of fat is in your blood stream. Elevated triglyceride levels may result in the hardening of your arteries or the development of pancreatitis. It will also dramatically increase your risk of heart attack, heart disease, and stroke. It has become common knowledge in the medical world that fasting triglycerides (how much of them are in your blood after fasting overnight) is a strong indication of potential heart disease.

While many people believe that eating a lot of fat will result in elevated triglycerides, it is really carbohydrates that are the culprit; especially in the form of simple sugar. Cutting carbs results in the dramatic decrease of blood triglycerides, which is the exact opposite result of low- fat diets.

5. Improved Levels of HDL Cholesterol

Not many people know that cholesterol comes in two forms: LDL and HDL. HDL, high density lipoprotein, is known as the "good" cholesterol. LDL and HDL direct the lipoproteins that transport cholesterol through the bloodstream. LDL actually transports the cholesterol from the liver to the rest of your body, but HDL carries it away from the rest of the body towards the liver to be reused or disposed of. The more elevated your HDL cholesterol levels are, your risk of heart disease is drastically lowered. The most efficient method of improving your HDL cholesterol levels is eating a low- carb, high- fat diet. HDL levels may only increase moderately or even go down when consuming a low- fat diet.

6. Decreased Blood Sugar Levels and Insulin Levels: In Relation to Individuals with Type 2 Diabetes

Type 2 diabetes is somewhat of an epidemic this day and age: the rising child obesity rates and poor eating habits of adults has resulted in an increase of this condition throughout the population. When we consume carbohydrates, the molecules are broken down into simple sugars, like glucose), within the digestive tract. Once broken down, the glucose enters the bloodstream and results in elevated blood sugar levels. However, high blood sugar levels are extremely toxic. Therefore, your body responds by producing the hormone insulin. Insulin communicates to your cells that there is too much glucose and they need to bring it down by either burning it or storing it.

Individuals who are health have a quick insulin response, which minimizes the blood sugar spike to prevent too much glucose from harming our bodies. However, millions of people suffer from major problems with responding to glucose spikes. Those with type 2 diabetes suffer from insulin resistance; when their cells do not recognize the insulin and therefore have a more difficult time lowering the blood sugar levels using your cells. It is crucial that your body produces enough insulin after meals to quickly lower your blood sugar; so patients with type 2 diabetes will inject even more insulin into their bodies after eating.

Cutting out carbohydrates improve your body's response to glucose spikes by eliminating the need for so much insulin. Therefore, both blood sugars and insulin dramatically decrease. In fact, keeping to a strict low/ no- carb diet will cure type 2 diabetes altogether within just a few months. However, if you are taking blood sugar- lowering medication, you should consult your doctor before making changes to your diet in order to prevent hypoglycemia (dangerously low blood sugar.

7. Your Blood Pressure Will Go Way Down

Hypertension, or elevated blood pressure, is not only a symptom of many diseases, but also a risk factor for developing new conditions. Such ailments include heart disease, heart attack, stroke, thyroid issues, diabetes, kidney disease, kidney failure, and many other diseases. Low carb diets are one of the most effective methods of quickly reducing blood pressure, which will help decrease the risk of disease and help you live a long and happy life.

8. Extremely Effective for Treating and Curing Metabolic Syndrome

Metabolic syndrome is a condition that includes a variety of serious and even fatal symptoms, including:

- Obesity

- High blood pressure

- Elevated blood sugar levels

- Elevated triglyceride levels

- Low DLD cholesterol levels

Metabolic syndrome increases the individual's risk of stroke, heart attack, heart disease, and type two diabetes. However, all symptoms of metabolic syndrome improve drastically while on a low- carb, high- fat diet. Unfortunately, major health organizations continue recommending a low- fat diet for individuals with this condition, even though it does not address the fundamental metabolic issue that causes these serious symptoms.

9. Increasingly Improves the Function of LDL Cholesterol

Low Density Lipoprotein (LDL) is known as the "bad" cholesterol and counter opposite of HDL. This is due to the fact that individuals with higher LDL levels are more likely to suffer from a heart attack. Although this idea goes against what we have been lead to believe about LDL, scientists have found that LDL matters when it comes to our health; not all LDL proteins are equal. This means that the size of the LDL protein particles is important and plays a large role in the state of your health. Individuals whose LDL is mostly made up of small particles have a heightened risk of heart disease, while people with large particles have a lower risk.

It has been found that low- carbohydrate, high- fat diets increase the size of the LDL particles, as well as reduce the number of LDL particles that are flowing through the bloodstream.

10. Low- Carbohydrate Lifestyles Help to Improve Several Brain Disorders

While low- carb diets are beneficial for a number of serious diseases, one of the most valuable uses of sticking to a ketogenic diet is acting as a therapeutic factor for life- altering brain disorders. Glucose is necessary for the brain, however only some parts of the brain are able to burn glucose. This is why your liver will create glucose out of excess protein if you stop consuming carbohydrates. However, a large part of the brain can also utilize ketones; which, as you know, are created when your body's carb consumption is very limited. This amazing and natural function of the ketogenic diet has been practiced for decades to help treat children with epilepsy when medicinal treatment fails.

In a number of cases, the Atkins diet has even cured children of epilepsy. One study concluded that more than half of the children who were fed a low- carb diet had a more than fifty percent reduction in their seizure episodes, with sixteen percent of the kids being cured altogether. The success with the low- carb, high-fat diet in epilepsy patients has inspired doctors and researchers to study the relationship between a ketogenic diet and several other disorders; for example, Parkinson's disease and Alzheimer's disease.

Part 2:

Atkins
21- Day Meal Plan

Chapter 5: 10 No- Carb Breakfast Recipes

1. Bacon, Cheese, and Avocado Breakfast Fiesta

Ingredients

> ½ of a Medium- Sized Tomato
>
> 1 Oz. Water
>
> 1 Medium- Sized Spring Onion
>
> 1 Slices of Cooked Bacon
>
> 1/3 Cup of Shredded Monterey Jack Cheese
>
> ½ Small Jalapeno Pepper
>
> 2 tsp. of Butter
>
> 1 tsp. of Lime Juice
>
> ½ Avocado, sliced
>
> ½ tsp. of Cilantro
>
> 2 Large Eggs

Directions:

1. Start by preparing your homemade salsa. First, chop the tomatoes, spring onion, and jalapeno pepper.

2. Combine these ingredients in bowl with the cilantro and juice from the lime. Set aside for later.

3. In a separate bowl, beat eggs with water. Then, crumble the cooked bacon and set aside.

4. Liquefy the butter at medium heat in a pan. When the pan is coated with the butter, add in half of the egg mixture. Tilt the pan so that the bottom is evenly coated with the egg, then continue cooking until the egg is almost set.

5. Add in the remaining egg, bacon, avocado, and cheese on top of the cooked egg. Let the contents of the pan cook for approximately one minute.

6. Fold the omelet over itself so that the filling is covered. Allow the eggs to cook for another two minutes before removing the omelet from the pan.

7. Serve your omelet with the salsa and enjoy!

2. Baked Eggs and Vegetables

<u>Ingredients</u>

4 Small Asparagus Spears

1 Tbs. of Almond Meal Flour

4 Tbs. of Heavy Whipping Cream

4 tsp. of Parmesan Cheese

2 Large Eggs

A Clove of Garlic, minced

<u>Directions:</u>

1. Heat oven to 400 degrees and prepare a small casserole dish with extra virgin olive oil or baking spray.

2. Next, boil the asparagus for approximately two minutes, until the spears are tender – crisp. Then, drain the vegetables and run them under cold water. Pat the asparagus dry and place in the casserole dish.

3. Pour the heavy cream over top of the asparagus. Now, crack the two eggs on top over the spears.

4. Now, in a bowl, stir the almond flour, cheese, and minced garlic. Sprinkle the mixture over top of the eggs. Put into the oven and bake for six to eight minutes, depending on how you like your eggs.

5. Remove the dish from the oven and enjoy!

3. Ham, Egg, and Garden Vegetable Breakfast Blend

<u>Ingredients</u>

1 ½ Tbs. of Extra Virgin Olive Oil

1 Plum Tomato

2 Tbs. of Butter

½ Medium- Sized Onion, chopped

1 Tbs. of Basil

1 Medium- Sized Bell Pepper

2 Oz. of Ham

3 Large Eggs

1 Clove of Garlic, minced

Directions:

1. Begin by heating the olive oil in skillet on medium heat. Put the onion into the pan and sauté until they are soft. Next, add in the garlic and cook with the onion for approximately one minute.

2. Next, add the peppers and tomatoes into the skillet. Cover the pan and cook the vegetables for ten minutes, until the veggies have softened. Stir the contents of the pan occasionally.

3. Remove lid from pan and have vegetables to simmer until the sauce thickens, stirring frequently.

4. In a bowl, whisk eggs until blended. Then, in a separate skillet, melt butter to layer the bottom. Add in the eggs and basil, and then cook and scramble the eggs until curds form.

5. Add the vegetable mixture and ham into the eggs and stir the contents until the ingredients are mixed together.

6. Remove your breakfast from the pan and enjoy with salt and pepper!

4. Pepper Rings with Egg Filling

Ingredients

2 Tbs. of Shredded Mozzarella Cheese

½ of a Large Red Bell Pepper

2 tbs. of Extra Virgin Olive Oil

2 Large Eggs

Directions:

1. Slice bell pepper across the middle. Next, cut two 1- inch thick rings from the pepper. Carefully use a knife or spoon to remove the ribs and seeds of the pepper rings.

2. Next, put the pepper rings into a skillet with the extra virgin olive oil. Cook over medium heat.

3. Now, crack one egg into each ring and continue to cook until the egg whites are fully set. Do not flip the egg.

4. Sprinkle the shredded mozzarella cheese onto the eggs and cover the skillet. Allow the cheese to melt for one minute, and then season with salt and pepper. Enjoy!

5. Spicy Eggs and Yogurt

<u>Ingredients</u>

2 Large Eggs

1 Tbs. of Chopped Leek

1 tsp. of Lemon Juice

1/3 Cup of Full Fat Greek Yogurt

4 Tbs. of Chopped Scallion

½ Clove of Garlic, halved

½ tsp. of Oregano

¼ Cup of Spinach

2 Tbs. of Butter, divided

1 ½ Tbs. of Extra Virgin Olive Oil

1 Dash of Chili Powder

<u>Directions:</u>

1. Heat your oven to 300 degrees. Begin by combining the yogurt and garlic in a small bowl. Add in a sprinkle of salt, and then set aside.
2. Add one tablespoon of butter and the oil in a skillet and melt on medium heat. Then, add the scallion and leek into the pan and reduce the heat to a lower setting. Continue cooking until the ingredients are soft: approximately ten minutes of cooking time.
3. Next, heat to medium – high and add the spinach and lemon juice into the skillet. Cook the spinach until the leaves have wilted, stirring often.
4. Now, transfer the spinach into a separate skillet, leaving the liquid in the original pan. Then, use a spoon to make deep indentations in the middle of the spinach for the eggs.

5. Crack both eggs into each indentation, and then cook until the egg whites have set: approximately ten minutes.

6. In a pan, liquefy the last tablespoon of butter on medium heat. Add in the remaining unused ingredients and cook until the butter begins to foam.

7. Now, remove the garlic from the yogurt dressing and discard. Dollop the yogurt over the eggs and spinach, and serve with a drizzle of spicy butter. Enjoy!

6. New Way for Bacon and Eggs

Ingredients

1 ½ Oz. of Cream Cheese

1 Pinch of Thyme

2 Large Hard- Boiled Eggs

2 Slices of Bacon

Directions:

1. Heat oven to 400 degrees and coat baking sheet with olive oil spray.

2. Begin preparing the cream cheese filling by combining the thyme and cream cheese in a bowl. Cover filling and put aside for later.

3. Next, peel the hard – boiled eggs, then carefully slice them lengthwise.

4. Use a spoon to remove the yolks from the white halves and discard. Fill two of the egg white halves with the filling, and then use the remaining two to cover the filling.

5. Next, tightly wrap slice of bacon around each of the eggs. Then, place the bacon- wrapped eggs in the baking dish.

6. Bake eggs in oven for thirty minutes. Remove from heat and enjoy!

7. Low- Carb Pancakes

Ingredients

2 Large Eggs

½ tsp. of Cinnamon

2 Oz. of Full Fat Cream Cheese

1 tsp. of Sugar

1 Tbs. of Butter

Directions:

1. Simply combine ingredients with blender; pulse until smooth. Allow the batter to rest for a few minutes as the bubbles settle.
2. Heat the butter in a skillet on medium- high so that it melts as a coating for the bottom of the pan.
3. Next, pour ¼ of the pancake batter into the pan so that it forms the shape of a pancake. Cook until the underside of the pancake is golden brown. Then, flip the cake so that the other side can bake.
4. When the underside has turned golden, remove the pancake from heat and repeat the process until you have used up the rest of the batter. Enjoy!

8. Spinach and Feta Breakfast Quiche

Ingredients

3 Large Eggs

4 Oz. of Button Mushrooms

2 Oz. of Feta Cheese, crumbled

½ Clove of Garlic, minced

5 tsp. of Parmesan Cheese

¼ Cup of Mozzarella Cheese

5 Oz. of Frozen Spinach, thawed

Directions:

1. Heat oven to 350 degrees and prepare a small pie pan with olive oil spray.

2. Start by squeezing the spinach in a paper towel, to remove the excess moisture. Prepare the mushrooms by rinsing them, then thinly slicing them.
3. Place a pan on medium heat, and layer with olive oil spray. Add the mushrooms and garlic into the pan and sauté until mushrooms are soft: approximately 6 minutes.
4. Next, place the spinach into baking dish, followed by the mushrooms. Add the crumbled feta cheese on top of the mushrooms to create a third layer.
5. Beat eggs and parmesan. Then, pour mixture on into the baking dish.
6. Finally, top the quiche with mozzarella cheese, and then put in oven.
7. Bake the quiche for approximately forty minutes, until the top is golden brown. Then, serve and enjoy!

9. Coconut Chia Seed Breakfast Pudding

Ingredients

¼ Cup of Chia Seeds

2 tsp. of Honey

1 Cup of Full Fat Coconut Milk

Directions:

1. Simple combine seeds, honey, and milk in a small bowl. Then, place in the refrigerator overnight.
2. In the morning, remove the bowl from the fridge and enjoy the pudding with a side of your favorite berries.

10. Salmon and Egg Avocados

Ingredients:

2 Large Eggs

1 Avocado

Salt and Pepper

1 Oz. of Smoked Salmon

¼ tsp. of Chili Flakes

Directions:

1. Heat oven to 425 degrees and prepare a sheet with olive oil spray.
2. Slice the avocado in half, lengthwise. Then, remove the seed. Use spoon to remove some of the avocado flesh, so that the holes are big enough for an egg to fit in.
3. Place the avocado halves onto the baking sheet and use the strips of salmon to line the hollows.
4. Crack the eggs into a small bowl, and carefully spoon the yolks and some of the egg whites into the avocado halves.
5. Season your breakfast with spices, and then put in oven. Cook for approximately eighteen minutes.
6. Remove from oven, and then top with the chili flakes. Enjoy!

Chapter 6: 10 Crave- Worthy Lunches

1. Caprese Omega- 3 Salad

Ingredients

¼ Cup of Balsamic Vinegar

½ Cup of Cherry Tomatoes, halved

1 Tbs. of Brown Sugar

2 Oz. of Fresh Mozzarella

4 tsp. of Extra Virgin Olive Oil

1 Avocado, halved, seeded, and diced

2 Cups of Romaine Lettuce, chopped

1 Tbs. of Basil Leaves

1 Boneless, Skinless Chicken Breast, thinly sliced

Directions:

1. Start by preparing the balsamic reduction. Do this by adding the brown sugar and balsamic vinegar into saucepan on medium heat. Allow the sauce to come to a boil, and then lower heat halfway. Cook for approximately seven minutes, and then set aside to cool.

2. Next, in a separate skillet, heat the oil on medium- high heat.

3. Place the chicken breast into the skillet and cook until meat is finished cooking; flipping the chicken once. Allow the chicken to cool before chopping it into cubes.

4. Finally, add the romaine lettuce into a bowl, and add chicken and remaining ingredients. Pour the balsamic vinegar dressing on salad and gently toss. Enjoy!

2. Low- Carb Shrimp Salad

Ingredients

¼ Head of Cauliflower

½ Cucumber

¼ lb. of Raw Shrimp

2 tsp. of Extra Virgin Olive Oil

½ Tbs. of Lemon Zest

1 Tbs. of Chopped Dill

Directions:

1. Preheat your oven to 350 degrees and layer sheet with cooking spray. Begin preparing your salad by peeling and cleaning your shrimp. Additionally, remove the tails as well.

2. Place the shrimp onto the sheet and put into the oven. Cook for eight minutes, until the shrimp is opaque.

3. While the shrimp is cooking, cut the florets off the cauliflower and discard the bottom stalk. Carefully chop the florets into small pieces, then place in a microwave- safe dish.

4. Cook the cauliflower in the microwave for five minutes, so that it is soft, but not mushy.

5. Set aside the shrimp and cauliflower to cool. Then, peel and chop the cucumbers into small pieces.

6. Once cooled, slice the shrimp into halves lengthwise. Then, in a bowl, mix together the all of the ingredients, evenly coating the cauliflower and shrimp with olive oil and lemon juice. Enjoy!

3. Zucchini Protein Pasta

Ingredients

1 Tbs. of Extra Virgin Olive Oil

½ Cup of Cherry Tomatoes

1 Medium Zucchinis

¼ Cup of Sun- Dried Tomatoes

½ Lemon, juiced

½ Cup of Basil, chopped

½ Serving of Vegetable Pasta

1 Oz. of Grated Parmesan Cheese

1 Large Poached Egg

½ Tbs. of Toasted Pine Nuts

Directions:

1. Cook the vegetable pasta in correlation with instructions providing on the packaging. While you are waiting for the pasta to cook, finely dice the cherry tomatoes and transfer them into a bowl.

2. Add the sun- dried tomatoes, garlic, lemon juice, basil, and a sprinkle of red pepper flakes (optional) to the bowl. Then, set the tomato mixture aside and allow to rest for ten minutes.

3. Now, use a spiralizer to spiralize the zucchini to create long noodles that resemble spaghetti. Add the zucchini noodles and veggie noodles into a deep bowl and toss together with oil.

4. Top your pasta with your homemade tomato sauce and poached egg. Sprinkle parmesan cheese on top with the pine nuts, and enjoy!

4. Portabella Mushroom Burgers

Ingredients

2 Portabella Mushroom Caps, stems removed

1 Slice of Halloumi

1 ½ Tbs. of Balsamic Vinegar

1 Thick Slice of Tomato

1 Tbs. of Extra Virgin Olive Oil

Directions:

1. Heat grill to medium heat, and wash and dry your mushroom caps.

2. In a small shallow dish, use a fork to whisk the balsamic vinegar and extra virgin olive oil. Then, place the mushroom caps gill-side down into to the dressing.

3. Next, place the mushrooms on the grill and cook for approximately five minutes; until they start to sweat. Then, flip the mushrooms so that the other side grills for another three minutes.

4. Place the halloumi on the grill and allow to cook for two minutes on both sides, until the cheese is pliable.

5. Start assembling your burger, using the mushroom caps as the bun and the cheese as the patty. Lightly season the tomato and then place the second mushroom on top to create the sandwich. Enjoy!

5. Spaghetti- Inspired Squash Pasta

<u>Ingredients</u>

1 Spaghetti Squash

1 Cup of Kale

¾ Cup of Chickpeas, cooked

2 Cloves of Garlic, min

1 Tbs. of Extra Virgin Olive Oil

½ Cup of Toasted Hazelnuts

2 Tbs. of Parmesan Cheese

<u>Directions:</u>

1. Heat your oven to 400 degrees, and prepare a sheet with olive oil spray.

2. Begin by slicing your spaghetti squash in half lengthwise, then removing the seeds. Rub each half with half a tablespoon of olive oil on the inside of the vegetable.

3. Place the squash facedown onto sheet and put in oven for forty minutes.

4. As the squash is baking, prepare the filling. Start by washing the kale and removing the ribs of the leaves. Then, roughly chop the leaves into small pieces.

5. In a pan, heat oil and minced garlic for two minutes. Add in the kale and continue cooking until the leaves turn bright green and have just started to wilt.

6. Next, add the chickpeas into the skillet and cook until they are warm. Then, transfer pan from heat and put aside.

7. Remove the baking sheet from the oven and use fork to remove the insides of the squash to form strands of spaghetti. Transfer the strands into a bowl, and the mix the spaghetti with the kale mixture.

8. Serve your dish topped with hazelnuts and parmesan cheese. Enjoy!

6. Simple Cucumber Salad

<u>Ingredients</u>

>1 Medium Cucumber
>
>1 Pinch of Pink Himalayan Salt
>
>2 Tbs. of Rice Vinegar
>
>1 Tbs. of Toasted Sesame Seeds
>
>½ tsp. of Sugar

<u>Directions:</u>

1. Start by peeling the cucumber, and then slicing it in half lengthwise. Next, use a spoon to scrap out the seeds.

2. Use a knife or carefully slice the cucumber into thin slices. Then, use a double layer of paper towels to gently press the excess moisture from the cucumber slices.

3. In a bowl, mix sugar, vinegar, and salt until the sugar is dissolved.

4. In a medium bowl, toss the cucumbers, sesame seeds, and dressing until the mixture is well combined. Enjoy!

7. Broccoli and Feta Salad

<u>Ingredients</u>

>1 Cup of Broccoli Florets, finely chopped
>
>3 Tbs. of Feta Cheese
>
>½ Cup of Chickpeas, rinsed
>
>2 Tbs. of Full Fat Yogurt
>
>3 Tbs. of Chopped Red Bell Pepper
>
>½ Tbs. of Lemon Juice
>
>½ Clove of Garlic, minced

<u>Directions:</u>

1. Start by whisking the feta cheese, garlic, and juice from the lemon in a bowl until the mixture is well combined.

2. Next, add the broccoli, red pepper, and chickpeas into the mixture and toss until evenly coated. Enjoy!

8. Tuna Salad with a Twist

<u>Ingredients</u>

6 Oz. of Chunk Tuna, drained and shredded

¼ Cup of Mayonnaise

½ Cup of Canned Artichoke Hearts

1 tsp. of Lemon Juice

2 Tbs. of Chopped Olives

½ tsp. of Oregano

<u>Directions:</u>

1. For this recipe, all you need to do is mix the ingredients together in a bowl. Enjoy!

9. Squash and Cheese Lunch Cakes

<u>Ingredients</u>

2 Cups of Summer Squash, shredded, seeds removed

1 Large Egg

2/3 Cup of Shallots, chopped

1 Tbs. of Extra Virgin Olive Oil

2 tsp. of Chopped Parsley

4 Tbs. of Parmesan Cheese

<u>Directions:</u>

1. Heat oven to 400 degrees. Begin by whisking the egg in a mixing bowl, then adding the shallots, salt, pepper, and parsley to season.

2. Next, place the shredded squash on a kitchen towel and squeeze out any excess liquid. Then, place the squash and cheese into the bowl that contains the egg mixture and combine.

3. Heat oil in skillet on medium heat and place a quarter of the squash batter onto the pan. Gently pat down the squash so that it forms a small cake. Cook the cake until it is brown and toasted. Then, flip the cake and allow to cook until browned.

4. Remove the squash cake form the skillet and repeat with the rest of the batter.

5. Place all of the cakes onto the skillet and carefully transfer into the oven. Bake for approximately eight minutes, and then serve.

10. Simple Chickpea Salad

Ingredients

Ranch Dressing:

1 Shallot, peeled

1 Tbs. of Buttermilk Powder

1 Tbs. of White- Wine Vinegar

½ Tbs. of Dill

¼ Cup of Cottage Cheese

2 Tbs. of Mayonnaise

2 Tbs. of Coconut Milk

Salt and Pepper

Chickpea Salad:

1.5 Cups of Cherry Tomatoes, halved

4 Oz. of Chickpeas, rinsed

8 tsp. of Red Onion, chopped

2 Tbs. of Crumbled Feta Cheese

Directions:

1. Start by preparing the dressing. Place the shallot into food processor and process until thinly chopped. Then, add the mayonnaise, buttermilk, cottage cheese, and vinegar into the processor and process smooth.

2. Pour milk in processor as it is running, along with the salt, pepper, and dill.

3. Now, begin preparing the salad but simply combining all of the salad ingredients in a medium bowl. Drizzle dressing in the bowl with the salad ingredients until evenly coated. Enjoy!

Chapter 7: 10 Simple Weight Loss Dinner Ideas

1. Honey Broiled Salmon

Ingredients

    1 Scallion, minced

    ½ lb. Salmon Fillet, skinned

    1 Tbs. of Honey

    2 tsp. of Soy Sauce

    1 Tbs. of Ginger, minced

    1 Tbs. of Rice Vinegar

    1 Clove of Garlic, minced

    ½ tsp. of Toasted Sesame Seeds

Directions:

1. Preheat your broiler and prepare a sheet with olive oil spray.
2. Begin by whisking together the vinegar, ginger, soy sauce, honey, and scallion in a bowl, until the honey has completely dissolved.
3. Next, place the salmon fillet in a sandwich bag and add half of the sauce mixture to marinate the salmon. Seal the plastic bag and place in the refrigerator for fifteen minutes.
4. Once the salmon is finished marinating, place the fillet one to the pan and broil approximately four to six inches away from heat until fully cooked through. This will take about ten minutes.
5. Serve the salmon with a drizzle of the sauce, topped with the sesame seeds. Enjoy!

2. Buffalo Chicken and Artichokes

Ingredients

    1 Large Artichoke, trimmed and prepped

¼ Cup of Shredded Cheddar Cheese

1 Lemon, halved

4 Tbs. of Hot Sauce

¼ lbs. of Cooked Ground Chicken

1 ½ Tbs. of Butter

1 Tbs. of Flour

½ Cup of Coconut Milk

Directions:

1. Begin by bringing pot of water to boil. Then, add the artichoke and lemon to the water, and bring to simmer. Cover pot and let cook for thirty minutes.
2. When the artichoke is finished cooking, transfer from the pot to a kitchen towel to allow the water to drain.
3. Now, preheat your oven to 400 degrees and prepare sheet with spray. Place the artichokes onto the sheet and splay the leaves.
4. Use a spoon to add the ground chicken in between the artichoke layers.
5. Next, liquefy butter in saucepan on medium heat. Add flour and beat with the butter for one minute. In small amount, pour the coconut milk into the saucepan, whisking the mixture until thickened.
6. Remove the saucepan from the stovetop and stir in the hot sauce and cheese.
7. Carefully pour the cheese over top of the artichokes and put in oven for ten minutes. Remove from oven and enjoy!

3. Simple Taco Skillet

Ingredients

½ lb. of Ground Beef

1 Cup of Baby Kale

½ Yellow Onion, diced

Taco Seasoning

1 Bell Pepper, diced

½ Cup of Shredded Cheddar Cheese

½ Can of Diced Tomatoes with Chilies

1 Zucchini, diced

Directions:

1. In a medium pan, brown the beef and crumble. Then, drain the excess grease.
2. Next, add the peppers and onion into the skillet and continue cooking until both vegetables have browned. Then, add in the canned tomatoes, taco seasoning, and as much water as the seasoning packet instructions calls for.
3. Now, add the kale into the taco beef mixture and mix well. Add in the cheese and allow it to melt into the beef, stirring frequently. Once the cheese has melted, remove from heat and enjoy over a bowl of lettuce.

4. **Spinach and Artichoke Frittata**

Ingredients

3 Large Eggs

1 Shallot, diced

2 Oz. of Marinated Artichokes, diced

1 Tbs. of Extra Virgin Olive Oil

1 Clove of Garlic, minced

4 Broccoli Florets, chopped fine

1 Tbs. of Chives

½ Cup of Spinach

1 Green Onion, finely sliced

2 Tbs. of Feta Cheese

<u>Directions:</u>

1. Coat a skillet with the oil on medium- heat. Add the shallots and garlic into the pan, and sauté for two minutes.
2. Next, add the broccoli into the pan and continue cooking until soft. Then, add in the spinach and stir into the mixture until the leaves have wilted.
3. While the vegetables are cooking, whisk the eggs and chives together in a mixing bowl. Pour the eggs into the vegetables and stir together.
4. Now, add in the artichoke hearts and allow the frittata to cook until the eggs are almost set. Preheat your broiler to 500 degrees.
5. Reduce the heat of the stovetop to medium/ low and continue cooking for an another two minutes. Transfer the skillet to the oven and broil until the frittata is browned.
6. Serve your dinner with crumbled feta cheese and enjoy!

5. Enchilada Zucchini Boats

<u>Ingredients</u>

Sauce:

½ Garlic Clove

¼ Cup of Chicken Broth

½ Tbs. of Hot Sauce

Salt and Pepper

1/3 Cup of Tomato Sauce

A Pinch of Chili Powder and Ground Cumin

Zucchini Boats:

1 Zucchini

¼ Cup of Green Bell Pepper, diced

½ tsp. of Extra Virgin Olive Oil

2 Tbs. of Chopped Cilantro

¼ Cup of Green Onions, diced

1 ½ Tbs. of Water

4 Oz. of Cooked Chicken Breast, shredded

½ Tbs. of Tomato Paste

½ Clove of Garlic, crushed

A Pinch of Cumin, Oregano, and Chili Powder

¼ Cup of Shredded Cheddar Cheese

Directions:

1. For the sauce, coat a saucepan with cooking spray and sauté the garlic. Then, add in the chili powder, broth, tomato sauce, and cumin to the pan and bring to a boil.
2. Reduce heat and let sauce to simmer for about ten minutes. Then, set aside to use later.
3. Now, bring pot of water to boil and preheat your oven to 400 degrees. Prepare a baking dish with cooking spray.
4. Slice the zucchini in half lengthwise and use a spoon to scoop out the inside, so that the shell is ¼ inch thick. Roughly chop the removed flesh and transfer into a small bowl.
5. Place the zucchini halves into the boiling water. Cook the zucchini for one minute, and then carefully remove the halves from the pot.
6. In a skillet, heat oil on medium- low heat. Add the onion, pepper, and garlic into the pan and cook until the onions are translucent.
7. Next, add the zucchini flesh into the skillet with the cilantro, and cook for approximately four minutes. Add the spices, water, and tomato paste into the pan and cook for three more minutes.
8. Now, add the chicken to the skillet and mix with the contents of the pan for a few minutes.
9. Pour half of the enchilada sauce into the baking dish, and then place the zucchini halves onto the dish, with the cut side facing up.
10. Fill the hollowed inside of the zucchinis with the chicken mixture, pressing the meat into the vegetable until filled. Use the rest of the sauce to cover the filled zucchini halves, and then top with cheddar cheese.

11. Cover the baking dish with aluminum foil and place in the oven. Allow to bake for thirty minutes, and serve once the zucchini is cooked through.

6. Pizza Frittata

Ingredients

½ tsp. of Oregano

6 Large Eggs

3 Tbs. of Dry Red Wine

3 Tbs. of Extra Virgin Olive Oil

½ Cup of Half- and Half

½ Cup of Crushed Tomatoes

1 Cup of Hot Pepperoni, chopped

¼ Cup of Parmesan Cheese

3 Oz. of Shredded Mozzarella Cheese

1 Clove of Garlic, chopped

1 tsp. of Hot Sauce

1 Tbs. of Grated Onion

1 tsp. of Chopped Parsley

Directions:

1. Heat oven to 400 degrees. Begin by whisking the eggs, cream, hot sauce, and parmesan cheese in a bowl.
2. Next, heat ½ of the oil in a pan on medium- high heat. Add the eggs into the pan and move them frequently until they start to firm.
3. Place the skillet into the oven and bake for approximately seven minutes.
4. In a separate skillet, heat remaining oil on medium- high heat and add cook the garlic, onion, and oregano for three minutes. Pour the wine into the pan and slightly reduce the heat.

5. Add the tomatoes into the skillet and simmer for ten minutes, until the sauce has thickened.

6. Remove the skillet from the oven and pour the tomato sauce over top. Sprinkle with mozzarella cheese and place into the oven once again for ten minutes. Top your frittata with parsley and enjoy!

7. Classic Chicken Wings

Ingredients

> 1 lb. of Wings and Drumettes
>
> ½ Tbs. of Butter
>
> 1 Tbs. of Thyme
>
> 3 Garlic Cloves, crushed
>
> ¼ Cup of Hot Sauce
>
> For Dip:
>
>> ½ Cup of Greek Yogurt
>>
>> ¼ Cup of Blue Cheese Crumbles

Directions:

1. Heat oven to 375 degrees and prepare a baking sheet with cooking spray.

2. In a medium bowl, season the chicken with salt and pepper.

3. Over low heat, melt butter in pan. Add in the garlic and thyme, and let simmer for two minutes. Then, add in the hot sauce, stirring the ingredients together.

4. Pour the hot sauce mixture over the chicken and toss well to evenly coat. Let the wings marinate in the refrigerator for a half hour.

5. While the wings are marinating, begin making your dressing. Simply combine the blue cheese and yogurt together in a bowl, and refrigerate for later.

6. Place the wings and drummettes onto the baking sheet and transfer to the oven. Bake for thirty minutes. Turn the chicken over, and baste with more hot sauce. Then, bake for an additional twenty- five minutes.

7. Remove wings from oven and let to cool before serving with the blue cheese dip. Enjoy!

8. Easy Steak Rolls

<u>Ingredients</u>

½ lb. of Flank Steak

½ Cup of Green Beans

¼ Cup of Steak Marinade

¼ White Onion, sliced into strips

½ Red Bell Pepper, sliced into strips

1 Tbs. of Extra Virgin Olive Oil

<u>Directions:</u>

1. First, marinade your steak in a plastic sandwich bag for thirty minutes with the steak marinade. While your steak is marinating, preheat your oven to 350 degrees and prepare a baking sheet with cooking spray.
2. Next, heat a skillet over medium heat and heat the olive oil in the pan.
3. Slice the steaks in halves. Take a little bit of the peppers, green beans, and onion slices, and tightly wrap the steak slices around the vegetables. Use toothpicks to secure the wrap.
4. Now, add the steak rolls to the skillet and sear for one minute on all sides of the wrap.
5. Carefully transfer the steak rolls onto the baking sheet and place in the oven. Cook for ten minutes, and then remove from the oven. Enjoy!

9. Simple Stuffed Chicken

<u>Ingredients</u>

1 Boneless, Skinless Chicken Breast

2 Oz. of Fresh Mozzarella, sliced

3 Oz. of Roasted Red Peppers, sliced into small pieces

2 Basil Leaves

2 Tbs. of Parmesan Cheese

½ Tbs. of Italian Dressing

Directions:

1. Heat oven to 400 degrees, and prepare a baking dish with cooking spray.
2. Use a knife to butterfly the chicken, cutting the breast lengthwise with about ¼ of an inch from the other side.
3. Spread the chicken breast into the dish, so that you can stuff it. Use salt and pepper to season the chicken.
4. Simply layer the roasted red pepper, and mozzarella cheese onto one side of the chicken. Carefully fold the other half over top, tucking in the stuffed ingredients snuggly into the chicken.
5. Drizzling the Italian dressing over top of the chicken, then place the dish into the oven. Bake for thirty to thirty- five minutes, until the chicken is full cooked.
6. Remove chicken from oven, and turn on your broiler to a high setting. Add any remaining mozzarella cheese and parmesan cheese onto the chicken and place into the oven once more.
7. Broil until the cheese turned golden brown, then remove from heat. Enjoy!

10.   Cauliflower Rice

Ingredients

1 Cup of Cauliflower

2 tsp. of Soy Sauce

¼ Cup of Onion, chopped

¼ Cup of Baby Carrots, chopped

1 Tbs. of Extra Virgin Olive Oil

¼ Cup of Thawed Frozen Peas

1 Egg, beaten lightly

1 Green Onion, chopped

½ tsp. of Sesame Oil

½ Cup of Bean Sprouts

Directions:

1. Slice the bottom of the cauliflower off, and then cut the cauliflower into florets. Dry off excess water.
2. Place the florets into a food processor and pulse until you achieve the consistency of rice.
3. Next, heat half of oil in skillet on medium- high heat. Add in the onion and fry until it is light brown. Transfer the onions into a bowl and set aside for later.
4. In a small mixing bowl, whisk the egg with the sesame oil and soy sauce. Add a bit more olive oil into the skillet, then quickly scramble the eggs.
5. Transfer the scrambled eggs from the skillet to the bowl with the onion.
6. Add the rest of the olive oil into the skillet and place the cauliflower, green onions, carrots, bean sprouts, and peas in the pan. Stir fry the ingredients for three minutes, then reduce to a lower heat setting.
7. Add in more soy sauce if desired, then cover until the cauliflower is good all the way through. Add the egg and cooked onions into the skillet once more and allow the ingredients to cook together for two minutes.
8. Serve and enjoy!

Conclusion

I hope this book was able to help you to understand the Atkins diet, as well as feel inspired to begin the first phase right now!

The next step is to make the decision to create a better life for yourself by changing your eating habits. You can have the body of your dreams and the greatest health you are able to achieve just by following this intensive meal plan. Health is the most valuable gift you could ever give yourself.

Finally, if you enjoyed this book, please take the time to share your thoughts and post a review on Amazon. It'd be greatly appreciated!

Thank you and good luck!